1

Make Your Own Herbal Medicine

A Practical Guide on Herbs and How To Create Simple & Effective Herbal Cures

Disclaimer and Terms of Use:

Effort has been made to ensure that the information in this book is accurate and complete, however, the author and the publisher do not warrant the accuracy of the information, text and graphics contained within the book due to the rapidly changing nature of science, research, known and unknown facts and internet. The Author and the publisher do not hold any responsibility for errors, omissions or contrary interpretation of the subject matter herein. This book is presented solely for motivational and informational purposes only.

Table of Contents

Introduction

Herbs have been used ever since prehistoric times. People from all over the world use herbal medicine to cure everything from common colds to dangerous disease. Herbal medicine still falls under the category of alternative treatment, but many studies show that it is just as effective as some medicines in the market.

Herbs contain amazing properties that serve as effective treatments for various physical and mental conditions. Herbal medicine can be taken in the form of powder, tablet and even oil extracts.

While commercial medicine only has one active ingredient, herbal medicine has several active and useful ingredients. Herbalists often recommend taking a combination of herbs to increase their potency or to lessen the side effects.

The use of herbal medicine is also part of a holistic and healthy lifestyle. Herbalists recommend proper diet that includes the consumption of whole foods and restricting processed junk food. Regular exercise and stress management can also increase the potency of the herbal remedy.

Having your own arsenal of home remedies has its own advantages. You can always rely on these natural treatments before you try conventional medicine. Surprisingly, medicinal herbs are quite easy to find and you might already have them in your kitchen cabinet. You can make a variety of herbal remedies from a simple tea to healing salve that you can use all year round.

Benefits of Herbal Medicine

Herbal medicine has a lot of known benefits. Unlike commercial medicine, it does not interfere with the natural healing process. Here are some of the other benefits of herbal medicine:

Natural healing

Herbs do not impede the body's healing abilities. It can even enhance the healing mechanism of the body and speed up recovery. Herbs can stimulate the glands and trigger the release of hormones. The hormones can signal body parts to work or inhibit biological processes.

Lifestyle changes

Herbal medicine is often accompanied by special instructions that include dietary change or exercise. An overall healthy lifestyle can enhance the potency of the herb and allows the body to respond properly to the treatment. In addition, if one follows these lifestyle changes even after recovery, then it is possible for him to reduce chances of reoccurrence significantly.

Improved Immunity

Herbs can help strengthen your immunity. It fortifies the natural defense of the body against pathogens that can lead to disease and infection.

Metabolism and Nutrition

A strong immunity leads to better metabolism and absorption of nutrients. Most herbal treatments restrict the consumption of junk food during the time of treatment because it contains toxins and stimulants that can interfere with the healing process.

More Economical

Prescription drugs are very expensive so it is natural for people to look for alternative cures. Herbs may not be as fast acting as conventional medicines, but studies support that it is effective just the same.

Fewer Side Effects

The side effect will depend on the herbs used. However, herbal medicine has fewer side effects than conventional treatment. For example, St. John's Wort that is useful for depression has fewer side effects than prescriptive medicine.

It is good for more than one condition

Prescriptive drugs are only used to treat one health problem. Herbal medicine, on the other hand, can affect different parts of the body all at once. For example, Gingko can improve circulation while also being effective when it comes to enhancing memory.

Common Herbs That You Should Have

Turmeric

Turmeric is a popular seasoning for curry and other spicy dishes. It contains curcumin, which has strong anti-inflammatory properties that act similar to drugs and prevent pain and swelling of arthritis.

Turmeric can also prevent Alzheimer's disease and colon cancer. Clinical studies show that curcumin can reduce lesions in the colon. It also helps clear the brain of plaques that can lead to Alzheimer's disease.

As a general guideline, you can enjoy adding turmeric into your dishes whenever possible. If you want to use it for therapy, aim to consume 400 mg of curcumin extract thrice a day.

Cinnamon

True cinnamon is the bark of a small evergreen tree that is native to Sri Lanka. Cinnamon is famous for its sweet and spicy aroma that can engulf your senses. It is commonly added to pastries and even beverages. Studies show that cinnamon can successfully reduce blood sugar level by 10%.

Cinnamon has other benefits for people with type 2 diabetes since it can also reduce the risk of heart problems. Cinnamon has also been used in ancient culture to cure gastrointestinal problems and relieve urinary infections. It has great anti-bacterial properties that can help relieve cold and flu symptoms.

Rosemary

Rosemary was first cultivated in the Mediterranean Sea. Rosemary is an herb that can survive poor soil and windy areas. Rosemary is part of the mint family. It has been used for different purposes. It is popularly known as an antioxidant. It can help prevent oxidative stress that can lead to many diseases.

Rosemary is also popular as a powerful anti-carcinogen. Studies show that rosemary can decrease the size of tumors in the mammary glands by 76%. Rosemary is also a good memory enhancer. It can inhibit the breakdown of acetylcholine, which greatly affects memory and reasoning.

The herb also has antibacterial and antiviral properties. Rosemary can eliminate harmful bacteria while keeping good bacteria undamaged. The most common way of using rosemary is by adding it to dishes as a seasoning. You can also make tea using rosemary leaves.

Ginger Root

Ginger root is a medicinal herb used as a remedy for many conditions including nausea, indigestion, cold, poor circulation, menstrual cramps and travel sickness. Since ginger has warming properties, it can effectively improve circulation and even help lower high blood pressure.

Ginger has also been used to treat gastrointestinal problems and dyspepsia. Studies show that ginger can affect the gastrointestinal tract and boost the muscles in the stomach to prevent strong intestinal contractions.

You can also use ginger to reduce inflammation in the joints and muscle tissue. Some athletes take ginger powder or tea after working out to help their muscles recover. If you are going to use ginger for travel sickness, then it is better if you take it 30 minutes before you travel.

Holy Basil

Basil is a popular flavoring for food. It can help treat several conditions from inflammation to bug bites.

Basil is recognized as a natural antidepressant. It can affect the adrenal cortex and stimulate hormones to regulate stress. This is the reason why most people use basil to improve mood. Basil is also effective against diarrhea, fever, skin infection and intestinal parasites.

Basil contains an active ingredient known as E-Beta-CaryoPhyllene that is effective in treating bowel disease and arthritis. BCP can naturally prevent inflammation that is related to arthritis.

You can use basil in different ways. You can use the leaves as seasoning or you can rub them directly into the skin to stop the itching caused by bug bites. You can also brew basil into a tea or add it in aromatherapy.

St. John's Wort

St. John Wort is a potent antidepressant that can treat mild to moderate anxiety. It can be just as effective as prescription drugs, but without the side effects. St. John's Wort has melatonin that can regulate the natural sleeping cycle of the body. The herb can also help combat side effects of emotional disorder such as OCD, mood swings and premenstrual syndrome.

In laboratory studies, it is shown to reduce the effects of nicotine withdrawal. St. John's Wort is also used for its anti-viral effects.

St. John's Wort acts as an inhibitor so avoid mixing it with alcohol, contraceptive pills as well as anti-epilepsy treatment. Topical St. John Wort cream can make the skin more sensitive to sunlight.

Garlic

Garlic is one of the greatest herbs that you can use every day. Garlic contains enzymes known as allicin, which is a strong antibacterial comparable to penicillin.

You can use garlic as a natural antibiotic. It is also effective in detoxifying the body and boosting the immune system. Garlic stimulates the production of glutathione, which is a strong antioxidant.

Studies also suggest that garlic can prevent plaque buildup in the blood vessels and prevent blood clots. Blockage of blood vessels can lead to vascular disease, stroke and heart attack. Garlic is also useful as a dietary supplement for diabetes and can prevent common cold.

Crushed garlic offers the best benefits. Fortunately, adding garlic in your food is relatively easy since it also adds flavor to your dish.

Ginkgo Biloba

Ginkgo biloba is one of the oldest trees in the Earth. Chinese herbalists have been using it for hundreds of years and people in Germany consider it as a prescription herb.

Ginkgo biloba extract can help enhance oxygen circulation in the body, which has mental and physical benefits. It is notably effective in improving memory and concentration. The herbal extract helps reverse damage to the eye and may improve long range vision.

It also has its antioxidant properties that can improve the nerve cell functions and help the blood flow in the body. Recently, there have been many studies regarding benefits of ginkgo biloba against Alzheimer's disease. Doctors believe that the antioxidant properties of gingko helps in slowing down the effects of the disease and can drastically improve the living condition of the patient.

Ginseng

Asian ginseng has been used for over 5,000 years. Ginseng is a highly priced herbal medicine. It has been used to promote overall health and long life. It is also said to treat many conditions including tumors, internal degeneration, fatigue, diabetes and stress.

In Western herbal medicine, it can help strengthen the immune system and prevent flu and cold. The herb has also been promoted to increase the survival rate of patients who suffered cardiac arrest.

Ginseng is said to be more potent if it is combined with gingko biloba. Avoid consuming large amounts of caffeine and other stimulants while using ginseng since it can cause complications like nervousness and elevated blood pressure.

Licorice

Licorice root has antidepressant properties. You can use this herb as an alternative to St. John's wort. This herb has many practical uses such as relieving asthma, athlete's foot, cold sores, gout, viral infection, liver problems and heartburn.

Licorice contains flavonoids and estrogen. Its main therapeutic compound, glycyrrhizin, provides many benefits for the body and can prevent the breakdown of adrenal hormones.

Licorice can cure ulcer because it is capable of lowering acid levels in the stomach. It can also be used to treat spasms and irritation on the digestive tract. Licorice is also effective in boosting the immune system by increasing the levels of interferon in the body that attacks the viruses.

Licorice eases congestion by thinning out the mucus in the airways. Licorice helps relax the bronchial tubes and sooth sore throat.

Marigold/ Calendula

Marigold or calendula has been used as a medicine for many centuries. It was traditionally used to treat minor injuries from warts, sunburn and sprains. It was also one of the first herbs that have been used to treat conjunctivitis and other eye inflammation.

Calendula has a high concentration of flavonoids that act as strong antioxidants in the body. It can help protect the cells from free radicals and oxidative stress. Calendula is also known to promote healing and reduce inflammation.

Creams that have calendula extract are good for the skin. It can help reduce acne and rashes. It also has strong antifungal benefits so it is effective against athlete's foot, Candida and ringworm. Compressed calendula blossoms can help reduce various veins.

Echinacea Purpurea

Having Echinacea in your medicine cabinet during the cold and flu season is advantageous especially if you are prone to contacting these illnesses on a regular basis. It is one of the best natural treatments for common cold.

Echinacea stimulates the immune system to fight all kinds of infection. Unlike antibiotics that target the bacteria directly, this herb makes your immune cells more efficient in attacking the bacteria. It also increases anti-tumor cells and stimulate tissue growth for wound healing.

Although Echinacea was traditionally used for internal problems, many use it at present for external application. It is also effective in slowing down the growth of bacteria and helps in the healing process.

Make your Own Herbal Recipes

Making your herbal treatment is not as difficult as it seems. After gathering herbs, you can create your own cough medicine, vapor rub and concoct treatment for various ailments. Making your own herbal recipes is also cheaper than buying commercial drugs.

You can also easily grow your own herbs. One of the advantages of having an herbal garden is that they are easy to grow. Even if you choose not to buy your own herbs, most of the ingredients for herbal remedies are readily available in herbal and food stores.

No Flu Tea

Natural treatments for flu and cold have been more like a family recipe that is passed down from one generation to another. This recipe makes a hot beverage that can help relieve cold symptoms.

Ingredients:

2 cups chicken stock

1 tsp cinnamon

2 whole cardamom pods

6 garlic cloves, minced

1 tsp turmeric

3 black peppercorns

Instructions:

Pour the chicken stock into a small pot. Add the remaining ingredients then stir to combine. Simmer the mixture for 7 minutes. Strain the liquid and pour into a mug. Consume while it is still warm.

Simple Cold Remedy

This is a natural cold remedy that is perfect to drink during a cold winter day. This warm tea can also help boost your immune system and improve brain activity to give you a jumpstart in the morning.

Ingredients:

2 lemon slices

1 tsp grated ginger

1 tsp cinnamon powder

Instructions:

Pour boiling water in your mug. Add the ginger and cinnamon powder. Stir to combine the ingredients. Add the lemon slices. Let it seep and cool for 2-5 minutes before drinking.

Migraine Relief Herbal Tea

Soothe headache and migraine using natural herbs. This tea may taste differently from the one you are accustomed to, but it is effective in relieving pain.

Ingredients:

4 parts chamomile flowers

2 parts feverfew

1 part passion flower

3 parts lemon balm

1 part skullcap

1 inch ginger root

Instructions:

Measure the herbs and combine in a large bowl. Transfer in a tea pot and brew. Let it boil then strain. Pour in a mug. Drink as usual.

Ginger Basil Tea

A cup of therapeutic tea can help ward off cold and cough during the winter season. Ginger and basil also have invigorating effects to your body and mind. The taste of ginger is predominant in the tea, but with a subtle basil aftertaste.

Ingredients:

½ tsp ginger, grated

4 basil leaves

2 cups boiling water

Instructions:

Place the ginger and basil in a teapot of mug or hot water. Brew for 5 minutes. Crush the basil leaves to release more of its flavor. Strain the liquid in a mug then serve.

Ginseng Soda

This is a great recipe to try if you want to make an alternative to commercial energy drinks and soda. The recipe is also straightforward and simple.

Ingredients:

¼ cup organic sugar

1 tbsp agave nectar

1 cup water

1 tbsp ginseng, powdered

1 tsp vinegar

Instructions:

Boil the water in a pot. Add the sugar and stir until it dissolves. Turn off the heat and let it cool for 3 minutes then add the ginseng powder, agave nectar and vinegar. Stir the mixture. To serve, add ¼ cup of the syrup to 1 ¼ cup of seltzer water. You can add honey if you want it sweeter.

Gingko Leaf and Ginseng Tea

Gingko and ginseng are among the best herbal remedies when paired together. They can boost the immune system and improve circulation. The tea can also help improve your memory.

Ingredients:

1 cup water

1 tsp ginseng, grated

5 gingko leaf

Instructions:

Place the leaves and grated ginseng in a bowl. Pour hot water and cover. Let it seep for 5 minutes. Strain the liquid into a cup and enjoy.

Rose and Calendula Cream

Use this cream to soften your skin and to prevent dryness. It is perfect to use right after washing dishes or tending your garden. A small amount will go a long way and you can also give this away as a gift.

Ingredients:

10 g or 2 tbsp grated beeswax

1 tsp aloe vera

10 drops rose essential oil

60 ml calendula infused oil

30 ml rose water

1 tsp vitamin C powder

Instructions:

Combine the oil and beeswax in a bowl. Set it in a Dutch oven until the wax melts. Remove from the heat then add the 40 ml rose water. Heat the rosewater in a small pot. The oil mixture and rose water should have similar temperature. Add the rose water to the oil gently. Whip the mixture constantly until the mixture thickens into a cream. Add the Aloe Vera, vitamin C powder and rose oil. Whisk the mixture again then scoop into a clean container. The vitamin C acts as a preservative so you can store it at room temperature.

Rosemary- Lemon-Eucalyptus Vapor Rub

Making your own vapor rub is a fun, economical and effective way to clear nose and chest congestion. Commercial vapor rubs contain crude oil that can be toxic especially to young children. This natural remedy is safer to use.

Ingredients:

4 tsp beeswax, grated

7 tbsp coconut oil

3 tbsp mango butter

20 drops rosemary essential oil

20 drops eucalyptus essential oil

20 drops lemon essential oil

Instructions:

Place the coconut oil, mango butter and beeswax in a glass bowl. Set it in a double broiler. Stir the ingredients until combined. Turn off the heat then add the essential oils. Pour in a small jar. This vapor rub can last for up to one year.

Herbal Cough Syrup

Herbal cough syrup can sooth your throat and relieve irritation. Honey has potent antibacterial recipe that can kill bacteria in the throat. Ginger and chamomile can reduce inflammation and sooth your muscles. Cinnamon boosts your immune system while the marshmallow root can relieve pain and promote sleep.

Ingredients:

¼ cup ginger root

¼ marshmallow root

¼ cup lemon juice

1 quart water

¼ cup chamomile flowers

1 tbsp cinnamon

1 cup honey

Instructions:

Pour water in a pan. Add the herbs. Stir the mixture then bring it to a boil. Simmer until the liquid is reduced by half. Strain the liquid to remove the herbs. Add the honey and lemon juice. Pour in a clean container and store in your refrigerator. Give 1 teaspoon for children and 1 tablespoon for adults. Take 2-4 times in a day until you feel better.

Healing Salve

Salves are wonderful to have in your medicine cabinet. It is useful for many conditions from diaper rash to insect bites. You can make your own healing salve from infused oil.

Ingredients:

1/2 cup St. John's wort

½ cup Echinacea leaf

½ cup yarrow flower

½ cup comfrey lead

½ cup Echinacea root

½ cup plantain leaf

½ cup calendula blossom

½ cup rosemary leaf

2 oz beeswax

1 tbsp vitamin E oil

Olive oil

Instructions:

The first step is to make an oil infusion. Use olive oil since it does not go rancid and it has great antimicrobial properties.

Place all of the herbs in a large jar. The herbs should fill the jar halfway through. Pour the olive oil on top. You do not want to fill the jar to the brim since the herbs can expand. Cover then place in front of a sunny window for 2-4 weeks. Shake it every day. Strain the oil using cheesecloth.

Pour the beeswax in a pot. Place it over heat until it melts. Add the oil then stir until ingredients are combined. Remove from the heat then add the vitamin E oil. Pour it into your container and allow it to set before using.

Cayenne & St. John's Wort Salve

Cayenne & St. John's Wort salve is great to have all year round. This tropical salve formula is useful in relieving muscle pain associated with extraneous physical activities and sports. You can also use this salve to warm your muscles during cold days.

Ingredients:

2 tsp organic cayenne powder

4 oz St. John's wort oil

½ oz beeswax

Instructions:

Prepare for a double broiler method. Combine the oil and cayenne powder in the bowl and stir until the mixture fully incorporates. Heat it up again, but be sure not to let it boil. Remove from the heat and let it seep for one day. Strain the mixture to remove the herbs. Pour the oil and beeswax in a double broiler then heat it until the wax melts. Pour in your glass container and allow it to cool.

Soothing Salve

Homemade soothing salve is made from medicinal herbs and oils that are rich in antioxidant and other healing properties. Unlike commercial salves, herbal creams do not contain chemicals and toxins that can harm your health.

Ingredients:

½ cup licorice root

½ cup calendula flowers

½ cup chamomile flowers

½ tsp palmarosa oil

½ tsp frankincense oil

32 oz olive oil

½ cup comfrey root

½ cup comfrey leaves

1 cup beeswax

½ tsp lavender oil

½ tsp chamomile oil

Instructions:

Pour the olive oil in a large pot. Add the comfrey roots and licorice. Stir the mixture and simmer for one minute. Check regularly to ensure that it does not boil. Add the calendula, chamomile and comfrey leaves. Stir and simmer for another minute. Strain the mixture in a bowl. Remove the herbs from the pot then return the strained oil to the pot. Place over low heat. Add in the beeswax and stir until the mixture melts. Remove from the heat. Add the essential oils. Scoop the mixture into containers and let it cool. This usually takes about 10-15 minutes.

Conclusion

There are many benefits of using herbs for common illness and disease. It can still surprise many people how herbs can provide such effective medicinal benefits because most people only think of them as culinary seasoning.

Aside from adding flavor to your dishes, herbs also boost your dishes' nutrient and medicinal properties. Use this book to create different herbal recipes that you can use every day. You can concentrate on using just one herb or mix a variety to create a concoction.

One of the best benefits of using herbal medicine is that you can use it in several ways. You can pulverize it and mix into your drink or brew it like a tea. Some herbs are even safe to cook and mix with food. Making your own medicine is like having your own pharmacy. You can create different products using medicinal herbs and customize them according to your needs and preference.

Enjoy this book?

Please leave a review below and let us know what you liked about this book by clicking on the Amazon image below.

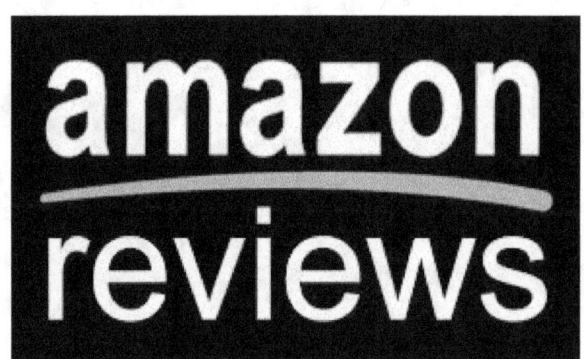

and click on Digital Orders.

The above link directs to Amazon.com. Please change the .com to your own country extension.